LARA ASHTON LEE

Facing Fifty Fearlessly

My Journey From Frustration to Fulfillment Through Sustainable Lifestyle Changess

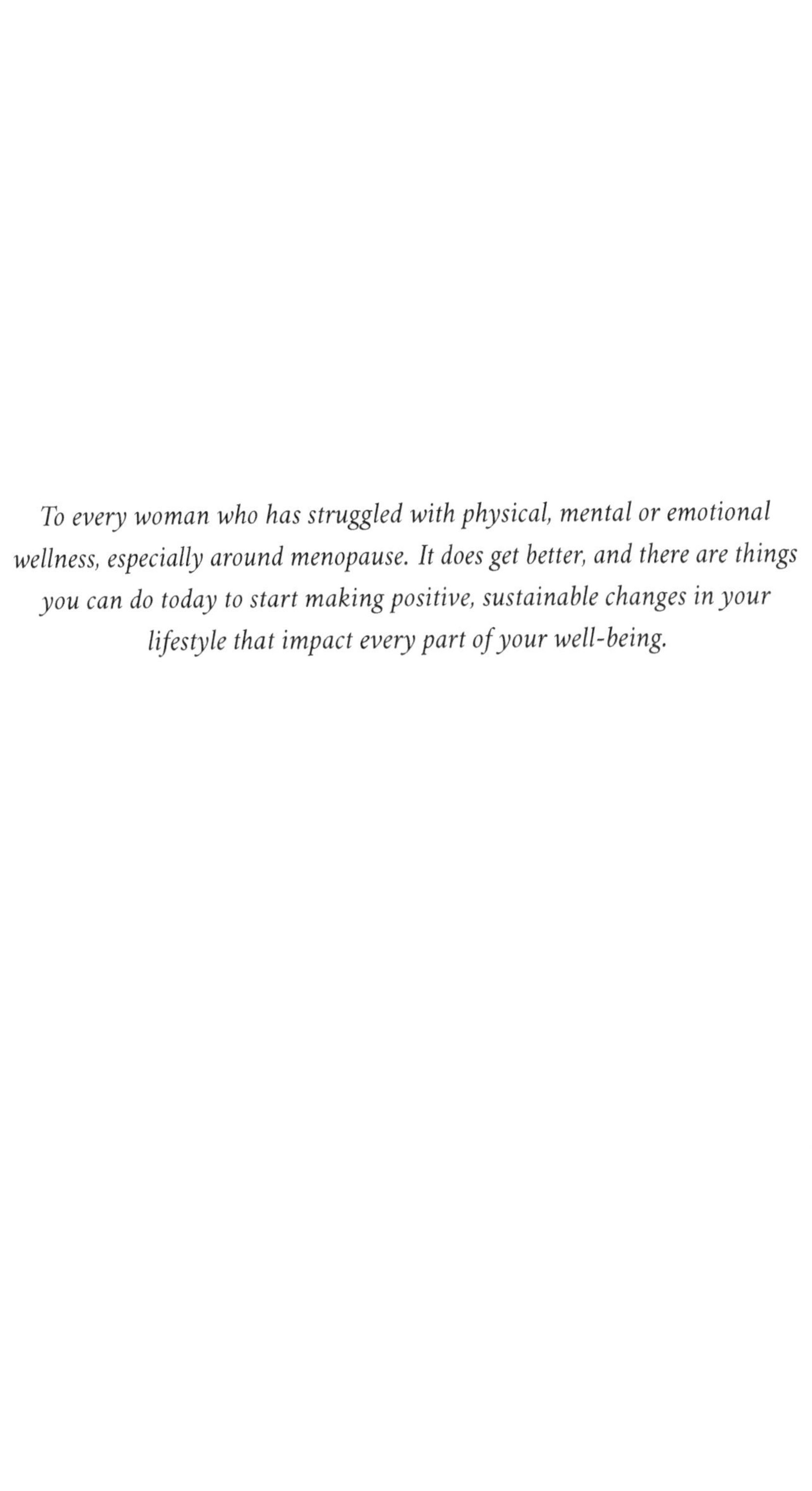

To every woman who has struggled with physical, mental or emotional wellness, especially around menopause. It does get better, and there are things you can do today to start making positive, sustainable changes in your lifestyle that impact every part of your well-being.

"And the beauty of a woman, with passing years only grows!"
—Audrey Hepburn

"So many women I've talked to see menopause as an ending. But I've discovered this is your moment to reinvent yourself after years of focusing on the needs of everyone else. It's your opportunity to get clear about what matters to you and then to pursue that with all of your energy, time, and talent."

— OPRAH WINFREY

Contents

1 The Beginning of My Journey   1

2 Initial Struggles and Realizations   3

3 Research and Discovery   5

4 Research and Discovery   7

5 The Importance of Gut Health and The Power of Probiotics   9

6 The Role of Fasting   12

7 Exploring Ketosis and Autophagy   15

8 Crafting a Sustainable Diet   19

9 Beyond Diet - Holistic Health Practices   23

10 Consistency and Continued Progress   26

11 Experimenting with Various Diets   29

12 Understanding Evolutionary Health   33

13 Psychological & Emotional Health   36

14 Building a Support System   39

15 Exercise and Movement   42

16 Overcoming Plateaus   45

17 Sharing Knowledge and Giving Back   48

18 Reflecting On Long-Term Sustainability   51

19 Embracing Change   54

20 The Emotional Rewards   57

21 Empowerment Through Knowledge   60

22 Building New Habits   63

23 Finding Joy in the Journey   66

24 Real Life Application   69

25 Addressing Skepticism and Misinformation   72

26 The Role of Healthcare Providers   74

27 Resources   76

1

The Beginning of My Journey

The Beginning of My Journey

I've been around the diet block. From Atkins to hCG to Jenny & WW (remember those acronyms?), I've tried them all. In some cases, the biggest outcome I achieved would be hunger and irritability. In many cases, I would have some initial hard-earned results, but in all cases, I would eventually wind up back where I started, or worse. The weight loss was almost always hard to attain, and harder to maintain. I have lost thousands of pounds over the years, but I've always ended up gaining as much as or more than I lost. It is a vicious cycle in every sense of the term, and it is exhausting.

The diet dance would always begin with enthusiasm, usually followed by a burst of energy, and positive feedback would sustain me for a bit, but inevitably the dance would end with a stumble offstage, disheveled and disheartened as the weight slowly came back, and along with it, frustration, and recrimination. My excess weight, that relentless partner, seemed to control my life. No matter how hard I spun, there was no way out.

But one day, armed with curiosity and a pinch of stubbornness, I embarked on a different quest. Research became my partner and friend. I dug into studies, dissected nutrition labels, and listened to the whispers of my gut (not literally—although, some days, it did have some things to say). And guess what? It wasn't entirely my fault. The diet industry had led me astray, like a GPS with a penchant for wrong turns.

Here's the revelation: Change doesn't require a grand sacrifice. No need to climb Everest or wrestle alligators. Pain? Nah, we're not masochists here. And neglect? Well, that's so last season.

So, I landed on a "program." Not a crash diet, mind you. This one felt like slipping into a cozy sweater—the kind that forgives your love for midnight snacks. Gradual progress became my anthem. Small steps, like breadcrumbs leading out of the diet labyrinth. Whole foods, not magic potions. Movement, not punishment. And rest? Oh, sweet rest, like a hammock swaying under a lazy sun.

I'm 49, and I started this journey over 100 pounds overweight. But guess what? The scale isn't my judge anymore. I've broken free from that cycle. Now my focus is balance, nourishment, and self-love. No more extremes. Just a steady groove toward health—one taco salad at a time.

So, my friend, if you're stuck in that diet dance, know this: It's not your fault. Change is possible. And the exit? It's right there, waiting for you to waltz through.

I've lost over 70 pounds without feeling deprived or controlled or starved or neglected. I'm excited to share what I've learned and hopefully help other women break free of the extreme diet and exercise cycle that has failed most of us, and find a new, balanced lifestyle that promotes health and well-being.

2

Initial Struggles and Realizations

My blood work and blood pressure thankfully have never been a problem, just the tendency to always gain weight steadily unless I was doing something extreme and unsustainable to keep it down. But just recently I had started having a bit of high blood pressure on occasion and my 'numbers' weren't as good as they used to be. It's a scary feeling when you realize your health metrics are starting to take a turn for the worse, especially as you get older.

I've struggled with my weight for literally my entire life, so I have always been painfully aware of the potential negatives that come with excess weight. There is no limit to the ailments which helpful people will blame on overweight - from aches and pains to depression to diabetes, heart disease and early death. Of course, the same helpful people will point out that its just a numbers game - burn more calories than you consume, and you will lose weight. Simple. Right? I wish it were that simple. I'm great at math. If I could MATH my way to a skinny waist, I'd be 105 pounds and I would live on a boat or a beach and I'd never have much clothes on. But that's a *whole* different book.

Anyway, back to simple math - so, if I put in less than I burn off, the weight will disappear.Either eat less or work out more.Easy. I also have a better than average amount of discipline, in spite of what my excess weight would tell you. So, I fully expected to have far more success than I did at everything I tried. Because I tried it all, from Jenny and WW, the memberships where you publicly weigh in every week or so, punishing yourself in front of your peers; to many of the different fads, rotation dieting, The Perfect Diet, Atkins, South Beach, hCG, the Zone. Then there were cleanses and detoxes and supplements, not to mention all the exercise fads. Everything did offer a small amount of early weight loss or energy boost, but it always seemed to require far more effort and return fewer results than it should. Add to that the fact that the rebound afterwards usually undid most of the progress. Frustration and self-recrimination to follow, naturally.

I like to think of myself as a reasonably intelligent person. I can learn. I enjoy learning, in fact. I prefer a documentary or an informative podcast to most other types of entertainment. It took most of my life, banging my head into the wall of weight loss misinformation, for me to decide enough was enough. Diet and exercise alone had not and would not solve my weight problem, and I was heading into scarier territory as I aged, with elevated blood pressure and worsening test results. I needed to find a different way, before it was too late. Education and information had always ben empowering for me in the past, so that is where I started in my quest for answers and solutions.

3

Research and Discovery

I did a lot of research, from books to medical journals to podcasts and even the ads my social media loves to throw at me to remind me I'm fat… I went down every rabbit hole I could find about health, aging, diet, wellness and any other keyword I could think of that might have useful information. I watched videos about exercise, how muscles work, and about digestion and gut biomes and the lymphatic system. I learned about water and electrolytes and bacteria. I tried to be as objective as possible as I read about so many different 'diets' from Atkins to keto, paleo, carnivore and snake diets, and all the way to vegan, whole food, the Zone, and of course, there's always cabbage soup or grapefruit to promote malnutrition. Through this extensive process, at some point, I stopped desperately looking for answers and just started trying to get a better understanding of what clearly doesn't work (diet and exercise) and what might.

Having largely given up on finding the right diet or exercise program, I just continued trying to learn. I watched videos and listened to podcasts. Once I wasn't as focused on the food, I was able to better focus on just what things were likely to promote better health. Without a specific diet, I just began trying to make better choices about what I bought and ate. I started trying intermittent fasting, because I knew from past experience that I always feel great at the beginning of a diet - so I figured I'd be safe trying to stretch the hours I wasn't eating a bit. It worked, and I felt good, so I started trying longer and longer intervals, with my goal being to get up to a week long fast. I'm not there yet - 72 hours has been my limit so far. Maybe by the next book.

In addition to the fasting, I started taking pre- and pro-biotics, and better supplements overall. During this time, I started noticing that my food cravings and choices were changing. A lot. I don't crave nearly as much food as I used to, and what I do want or crave are smaller portions of food that is healthier than I have gravitated toward for most of my life. This made me think - the last time I felt this in touch with my body was when I was pregnant with my children, who are all over 20 years old. I think our bodies know what we need, and I also think they try to tell us. The American diet is essentially completely anathema to our health and wellbeing. Portions at restaurants are crazy large, everything is processed or breaded, fried and gravied. We are among the most educated, and yet also somehow the most unhealthy people who have ever existed. Obesity is an epidemic, and it is steadily on the rise, especially among our children. And we're still telling them the same wrong things we were all told, that they just need to eat less or move more. If they just had the discipline, they could overcome their problem. It's not that hard, after all, right? I'm certain it is doing the same damage to their self esteem and self worth as it did mine.

I honed in on a combination of practices grounded in scientific research and validated by numerous success stories, but which also made logical sense to me. This was something that I had stopped doing, because weight and health had stopped making any sense so long ago I can barely remember.

4

Research and Discovery

I did a lot of research, from books to medical journals to podcasts and even the ads my social media loves to throw at me to remind me I'm fat… I went down every rabbit hole I could find about health, aging, diet, wellness and any other keyword I could think of that might have useful information. I watched videos about exercise, how muscles work, and about digestion and gut biomes and the lymphatic system. I learned about water and electrolytes and bacteria. I tried to be as objective as possible as I read about so many different 'diets' from Atkins to keto, paleo, carnivore and snake diets, and all the way to vegan, whole food, the Zone, and of course, there's always cabbage soup or grapefruit to promote malnutrition. Through this extensive process, at some point, I stopped desperately looking for answers and just started trying to get a better understanding of what clearly doesn't work (diet and exercise) and what might.

Having largely given up on finding the right diet or exercise program, I just continued trying to learn. I watched videos and listened to podcasts. Once I wasn't as focused on the food, I was able to better focus on just what things were likely to promote better health. Without a specific diet, I just began trying to make better choices about what I bought and ate. I started trying intermittent fasting, because I knew from past experience that I always feel great at the beginning of a diet - so I figured I'd be safe trying to stretch the hours I wasn't eating a bit. It worked, and I felt good, so I started trying longer and longer intervals, with my goal being to get up to a week long fast. I'm not there yet - 72 hours has been my limit so far. Maybe by the next book.

In addition to the fasting, I started taking pre- and pro-biotics, and better supplements overall. During this time, I started noticing that my food cravings and choices were changing. A lot. I don't crave nearly as much food as I used to, and what I do want or crave are smaller portions of food that is healthier than I have gravitated toward for most of my life. This made me think - the last time I felt this in touch with my body was when I was pregnant with my children, who are all over 20 years old. I think our bodies know what we need, and I also think they try to tell us. The American diet is essentially completely anathema to our health and wellbeing. Portions at restaurants are crazy large, everything is processed or breaded, fried and gravied. We are among the most educated, and yet also somehow the most unhealthy people who have ever existed. Obesity is an epidemic, and it is steadily on the rise, especially among our children. And we're still telling them the same wrong things we were all told, that they just need to eat less or move more. If they just had the discipline, they could overcome their problem. It's not that hard, after all, right? I'm certain it is doing the same damage to their self esteem and self worth as it did mine.

I honed in on a combination of practices grounded in scientific research and validated by numerous success stories, but which also made logical sense to me. This was something that I had stopped doing, because weight and health had stopped making any sense so long ago I can barely remember.

5

The Importance of Gut Health and The Power of Probiotics

In addition to the normal supplements that I have taken for years (fish oil, a multivitamin high in vitamin D, L-carnitine and glucosamine especially) I have added live pre- and probiotics. I happen to believe that this is among the most important things we need to do for our health. I can't overstate how important I have come to believe this is. I make sure that I am getting the most potent formulations that cover each part of the digestive system.

Gut Health: A Key to Overall Well-Being

The gut, often referred to as the gastrointestinal (GI) tract, is a complex system responsible for digestion, nutrient absorption, and immune function. Its health impacts various aspects of our well-being. When you consider the role that it plays in extracting the nutrients from our food as well as disposing of waste material, it is easy to see why maintaining a healthy gut is so important:

- Digestion and Nutrient Absorption: The gut breaks down food into essential nutrients (such as vitamins, minerals, and amino acids) that our body needs for energy, growth, and repair. Proper digestion ensures efficient nutrient absorption.

- Microbiome Balance: Inside the gut resides a diverse community of microorganisms—the gut microbiome. These bacteria, viruses, and fungi play a vital role in digestion, metabolism, and immune regulation. A balanced microbiome promotes overall health.
- Immune System Support: Over 70% of our immune cells reside in the gut. A healthy gut microbiome is kind of the front-line immunity responder, defending against infections and diseases.
- Mental Health Connection: The gut-brain axis links gut health to mental well-being. Imbalances in the microbiome may contribute to anxiety, depression, and cognitive function. Nurturing the gut can positively impact mood and stress levels.
- Reducing Inflammation: Chronic inflammation is associated with various health conditions, including heart disease, diabetes, and autoimmune disorders. A well-functioning gut helps prevent excessive inflammation.

Remember, a balanced diet rich in fiber, probiotics, and prebiotics supports gut health. I want to reiterate here the surprising role our gut plays in both our mental well-being and our immune system. As I was exploring different aspects of health overall, I kept seeing connections drawn between the brain and the gut, and between the immune system and the digestive system. Inflammation is another key concept that I keep running into in relation to its role in the complex system of our bodies.

I always encourage people to do their own research, and certainly consult your healthcare professional before doing anything significant that could affect your health, especially if you are dealing with anything serious, health wise. It is often good to ease into things, so as not to shock your system. I would say to use your best judgment and common sense, but that doesn't always work. Consult professionals wherever possible.

6

The Role of Fasting

Next, I have been incorporating fasting into my schedule, experimenting with different types of fasting. It has been a game-changer. Initially, I started with intermittent fasting, trying different intervals. I eventually worked my way up to an 18:6 interval, which significantly boosted my weight loss and kept it moving steadily. Recently, I have also been experimenting with longer fasts—24, 30, even 36-hour fasts. Each of these extended fasts kick-starts a significant drop in weight, makes me feel rejuvenated, and, I believe, helps in healing any damage caused by my previously sedentary lifestyle.

Fasting, a practice that dates back centuries and plays a central role in many cultures and religions, offers several health benefits. Let's explore these benefits, backed by scientific research:

Blood Sugar Control and Insulin Sensitivity:

- Intermittent fasting and alternate-day fasting can improve blood sugar control by reducing insulin resistance. This helps transport glucose efficiently from the bloodstream to cells, preventing spikes and crashes in blood sugar levels.

- Fasting may reduce risk factors associated with metabolic syndrome, which increases the likelihood of type 2 diabetes, heart disease, and stroke.

Inflammation Reduction:

- Chronic inflammation is linked to conditions like heart disease, cancer, and rheumatoid arthritis. Fasting can decrease inflammation levels.
- Intermittent fasting has been shown to significantly reduce C-reactive protein (a marker of inflammation) and improve overall health.

Heart Health:

- Some restrictive diets, including intermittent fasting, can benefit heart health by improving cholesterol levels and reducing inflammation.
- Fasting may also enhance cardiovascular function and reduce risk factors for heart disease.

Brain Function and Longevity:

- Theories suggest that periodic fasting may boost brain function and prevent neurodegenerative diseases.
- Fasting triggers autophagy, a cellular process that removes damaged components and promotes longevity.

Weight Loss and Metabolic Improvements:

- Fasting promotes weight loss by tapping into stored fat for energy.
- It can improve metabolic markers, such as insulin sensitivity and lipid profiles.

Remember, as with any significant change in your lifestyle, fasting should be approached safely and with guidance. Speak with a healthcare professional before starting any fasting regimen. I also recommend easing into anything new gently. It helps me by reducing any discomfort that could be caused, and makes it easier to adjust and be successful.

7

Exploring Ketosis and Autophagy

I f you search ketosis and autophagy, you'll discover some fascinating insights into the human body. For instance, one of the Nobel Prize Winners in the last decade was awarded for discovering the process of autophagy. Ketosis, or the production of ketones by the liver as a byproduct of fat metabolism, is equally interesting. Both processes have profound effects on the body, facilitating cellular repair and enhancing metabolic efficiency.

Ketosis

Ketosis is a metabolic state where your body shifts from using glucose (from carbohydrates) as its primary energy source to burning fat. The ketogenic (keto) diet intentionally induces ketosis by significantly reducing carbohydrate intake and increasing fat consumption. Here are the benefits of ketosis, supported by scientific research:

- **Weight Loss**: Ketosis promotes weight loss by utilizing stored fat for energy. When carbs are restricted, the body turns to fat stores, leading to fat breakdown and subsequent weight reduction.

- **Improved Blood Sugar Control**: Ketosis may enhance blood sugar management. By minimizing carb intake, it reduces blood sugar spikes and insulin resistance, potentially benefiting individuals with type 2 diabetes.
- **Increased Energy**: Some people experience improved energy levels during ketosis. Stable blood sugar and efficient fat utilization contribute to sustained energy throughout the day.
- **Better Cognitive Function:** Ketones, produced during ketosis, serve as an alternative fuel for the brain. Some studies suggest that ketosis may enhance cognitive performance and focus.
- Potential Anti-Inflammatory Effects: Ketosis may reduce inflammation markers in the body, contributing to overall health and disease prevention.
- **Epilepsy Management:** Ketogenic diets have been used since the 1920s to treat drug-resistant epilepsy in children. The diet's ability to reduce seizures remains a well-established benefit.

Remember, while ketosis offers advantages, it's essential to maintain a balanced approach and consult a healthcare professional before adopting any dietary changes.

Autophagy

Autophagy, a fundamental cellular process, plays a crucial role in maintaining cellular health and homeostasis. Let's delve into the details of autophagy and its significance, along with references to the Nobel Prize awarded for its discovery.

What Is Autophagy?

- Autophagy (from the Greek words "auto" meaning self and "phagy" meaning eating) is a process by which cells break down and recycle their own components.

- During autophagy, cellular organelles, proteins, and other structures are engulfed by specialized vesicles called autophagosomes.
- These autophagosomes fuse with lysosomes, where their contents are degraded and recycled.

Mechanisms of Autophagy:

- **Macroautophagy**: The most well-known form of autophagy. It involves the formation of autophagosomes that engulf cytoplasmic material.
- **Microautophagy**: Direct engulfment of cytoplasmic components by lysosomes.
- **Chaperone-Mediated Autophagy (CMA)**: Specific proteins are selectively targeted for degradation within lysosomes.

Why Is Autophagy Important?

- **Cellular Quality Control**: Autophagy removes damaged organelles, misfolded proteins, and other cellular debris, preventing their accumulation.
- **Energy Metabolism**: During nutrient scarcity (such as fasting), autophagy provides an alternative energy source by breaking down cellular components.
- **Aging and Longevity**: Dysfunctional autophagy is associated with aging and age-related diseases.
- **Immune Response**: Autophagy contributes to antigen presentation and immune surveillance.

Nobel Prize and Yoshinori Ohsumi:

- In 2016, **Yoshinori Ohsumi**, a Japanese cell biologist, was awarded the **Nobel Prize in Physiology or Medicine** for his groundbreaking discoveries related to autophagy mechanisms.
- Ohsumi's work focused on understanding autophagy in yeast cells. His research revealed essential genes involved in autophagy and provided insights into its regulation and significance.

In summary, autophagy is a fundamental process that maintains cellular health, promotes longevity, and adapts to changing environmental conditions. Yoshinori Ohsumi's contributions were pivotal in unraveling the mysteries of autophagy, leading to the prestigious Nobel recognition

8

Crafting a Sustainable Diet

Transitioning from fasting, my diet is centered around consuming foods that are as fresh and unprocessed as possible. While I do occasionally order in, I focus on moderation and quality in what I eat, including the occasional indulgence in potatoes, pasta, or sweets. Intermittent fasting and improving my gut health have remarkably adjusted my cravings, tastes, and appetite, which has become a crucial aspect of making this lifestyle sustainable.

My diet is largely just trying to find the easiest, most affordable yet freshest and least processed foods as possible. Some days the healthiest food I can find and stand to eat comes wrapped in paper with fries on the side. And if I really want it, I get it. I try to enjoy it as much as possible while eating as little as possible. Other days, I actually want a healthy salad.

Until a few years ago, I did not would not have believed that a person could actually enjoy a leafy salad unless it came with steak or fried chicken, loads of dressing, plus cheese, croutons and of course, maybe a little bacon. These days, if I eat a salad, I want that salad, and I will enjoy it. After almost 50 years of being me, living in my body and knowing what I like, my tastes and cravings are truly very different than they used to be. The only changes that I madethings that changed prior to my appetites changing were the intermittent fasting and probiotics. I think that by giving my body even a small chance at working at peak efficiency after almost 50 years of using it wrong, it has actually started to work better, and I think that my appetites and cravings are a sign of that.These things also make sense from an evolutionary standpoint. If I were around when folks were carrying clubs and living in caves, I'm pretty sure I would be more of a hunter than a gatherer. It makes way more sense in terms of time invested, calories spent and calories 'harvested.' I'm sure there was a good amount of berry eating going on, mainly because berries are wonderful, but I do not think that there were many vegans living in caves. My logic tells me that we would have had regular hunting parties getting us good old fashioned protein as our main source of calories. If the hunting wasn't going well, there would be the berries to fall back on, but I just don't see Fred Flinstone as much of a mushroom, nut and spinach guy. Also, don't forget that quite literally everything they ate back then was non-GMO, organic, and containing zero preservatives. None of it was processed, or fat or sugar free. As far as I know, everyone agrees that there was very little obesity during the last ice age, despite them not having access to the latest prescription weight loss drugs or gastric bypass surgery. Imagine that.

A whole foods diet emphasizes consuming minimally processed foods in their natural state. Here's why it's beneficial and some tips to get started:

What Is a Whole Foods Diet?

- A whole foods diet involves choosing foods that are **minimally processed**.
- Key components include fresh fruits, vegetables, nuts, seeds, oils, and whole grains.

- It doesn't necessarily require becoming a vegetarian or vegan; meat and dairy can be part of it in moderation.

Benefits of Whole Foods:

- **Nutrient-Rich**: Unprocessed foods are naturally rich in essential vitamins, minerals, antioxidants, and fiber.
- **Low in Saturated Fat and Sodium**: Whole foods tend to have lower levels of unhealthy fats and salt.
- **Health Outcomes**: Studies link plant-based whole foods to reduced risks of heart disease, diabetes, hypertension, obesity, and certain cancers.

Tips for Starting a Whole Foods Diet:

- **Gradual Transition**: Begin by planning at least one fully vegetarian meal per week. Gradually increase the frequency.
- **Spice It Up**: Experiment with herbs and spices to add flavor to plant-based meals.
- **Variety**: Explore different whole foods—fruits, veggies, legumes, whole grains—to keep meals interesting and nutritious.

Remember, a whole foods diet promotes health, longevity, and environmental sustainability. Prioritize fresh, unprocessed options whenever possible!

I do want to mention here that you can go on a whole foods diet without breaking the bank. There are many different ways to adapt whatever your diet is right now and work on making fresher, healthier and less processed food choices. One recommendation is to only shop around the outside of the grocery store, from produce and fresher bakery items through meats and dairy, skipping many of the boxed, processed, canned and frozen foods. Not all foods found in cans or the freezer section are unhealthy. The nutrients have not all been removed from canned foods, and frozen fruits and vegetables are not necessarily less healthy than their fresh counterparts. In a perfect world, we would all be able to afford fresh, organic, non-GMO, cage free, free range, wild & unfarmed foods. We do not live in such a utopia, and food costs have only been rising more and faster, and the geopolitical climate does not look good for that to change in the foreseeable future. What matters is that you do what you can. Opt for less processed and fresher where you can. Be informed about what you are eating and try to avoid ingredients you can't pronounce or identify. If you are deliberate and aware and proactive about what and how and when you eat, it is easier than you think to make a difference.

- Harvard T.H. Chan School of Public Health: Their article on "The Nutrition Source" provides evidence-based guidance on healthy eating, emphasizing whole foods.
- World Health Organization (WHO): The WHO's guidelines on "Healthy Diet" emphasize whole foods and their impact on health.
- American Heart Association (AHA): The AHA's recommendations on "Diet and Lifestyle Recommendations" highlight the importance of whole foods for heart health.

Remember to explore these sources for more detailed information.

9

Beyond Diet - Holistic Health Practices

In addition to diet and fasting, I am also incorporating other health-promoting practices such as meditation, drinking hydrogen water, and using specific types of salts. Over time, I've found these practices not only complement my weight loss efforts but also enhance my overall well-being. Meditation helps manage stress, while hydrogen water and specialized salts provide additional physiological benefits. I mention this here, because I believe these things are helping me to be successful by promoting both physical and mental well-being. Our bodies are a complex system, and we can't have overall health and wellness if we are neglecting some parts of our bodies while focusing too much on other areas.

Meditation:

- Meditation is a powerful practice that has been used for centuries to promote mental and emotional well-being. It involves focusing your mind and eliminating distractions, which can reduce stress, anxiety, and improve overall mental clarity.
- Research suggests that regular meditation can positively impact var-

ious aspects of health, including blood pressure, immune function, and even pain management.
- Sources: Harvard Health Publishing

Hydrogen Water:

- Hydrogen water (also known as hydrogen-rich water) contains dissolved molecular hydrogen (H_2). It has gained attention for its potential health benefits.
- Some studies suggest that hydrogen water may act as an antioxidant, reduce inflammation, and improve exercise performance.
- However, more research is needed to fully understand its effects and optimal dosage.
- Sources: National Institutes of Health (NIH)

Specialized Salts:

- Certain types of salts, such as Baja Gold, Himalayan Ppink salt or even generic sea salt, are considered healthier alternatives to regular table salt (sodium chloride).
- These salts contain trace minerals that may offer additional health benefits, including better electrolyte balance and improved hydration.
- However, moderation is key, as excessive salt intake can still be harmful to health.
- Sources: Cleveland Clinic

Remember that individual responses to these practices can vary, and it's essential to consult with a healthcare professional before making significant changes to your routine. Incorporating a holistic approach to health, including diet, exercise, and stress management, can contribute to overall well-being.

10

Consistency and Continued Progress

My journey has taught me that consistency is key, and small, incremental changes can lead to significant, lasting results. Since beginning this approach, I've lost 65 pounds in under six months and continue to lose weight. Moreover, these changes have positively impacted various aspects of my life, from my energy levels to my mental clarity and overall mood.

Consistency is indeed the bedrock of achievement in any endeavor. Whether you're pursuing personal growth, professional goals, or creative projects, maintaining a steady and unwavering effort is essential. Let's explore why consistency matters and how it leads to success:

Building Habits:

- Consistency helps transform actions into habits. When you consistently engage in a specific behavior, it becomes ingrained in your daily routine.
- Habits are powerful because they operate on autopilot. Imagine waking up early every day to exercise—it becomes second nature, and you're more likely to stick with it.

Compound Effect:

- The compound effect, popularized by Darren Hardy, emphasizes that small, consistent actions yield significant results over time.
- Think of it as a snowball rolling down a hill. Initially, it's tiny, but as it accumulates more snow (consistent effort), it grows exponentially.

Skill Mastery:

- Consistent practice leads to skill mastery. Whether you're learning an instrument, a language, or a sport, regular practice hones your abilities.
- The 10,000-hour rule (from Malcolm Gladwell's "Outliers") suggests that expertise emerges after approximately 10,000 hours of deliberate practice.

Mental Conditioning:

- Consistency trains your mind. It reinforces discipline, resilience, and focus.
- When faced with obstacles or setbacks, consistent individuals persevere because their mental conditioning propels them forward.

Trust and Reliability:

- Consistency builds trust. People rely on those who consistently deliver—whether it's meeting deadlines, providing quality work, or showing up consistently.
- Trust is the currency of relationships, both personal and professional.

Overcoming Plateaus:

- Progress isn't always linear. There are plateaus where it seems like nothing is changing.
- Consistency during plateaus is crucial. It's when breakthroughs occur—often unexpectedly.

Long-Term Vision:

- Consistency aligns with long-term vision. Success rarely happens overnight; it's the result of persistent effort.
- Picture a marathon runner—each step contributes to crossing the finish line.

In summary, consistency isn't flashy or glamorous, but it's the quiet force that propels you toward your goals. So, whether you're writing a novel, building a business, or improving your health, remember that consistency is your steadfast companion on the journey to success.

11

Experimenting with Various Diets

One of the most enlightening parts of this journey has been experimenting with different dietary approaches. I've considered trying the carnivore diet, which emphasizes meat and animal products, and contrastingly, a vegan diet, which focuses on plant-based foods. Both have unique benefits, and by researching and trying out elements of each, I've learned a lot about how different foods and dietary patterns affect my body. I've also learned better how to listen to my body and how to make small adjustments, and give them some time to take effect before determining if something does or doesn't work for me. At times, I have kept food diaries, trying to see if I could pinpoint positive or negative impacts from different foods or supplements or whatever variable I am looking at.

Every time I have been disciplined and deliberate in what I am doing for my health, I have learned something. Sometimes, the only thing I learned is that I don't like how I feel on certain diets or supplements. Other times, I have noticed increased or decreased energy levels or irritability or good or bad effects on my sleep or digestion. I have never felt like it was a waste of time or effort to collect information. Sometimes it is more effort than I am willing to put into food or exercise diaries, especially if it is during holidays or vacations or other extremely busy times, but still never a waste of time. I would encourage anyone who is interested in changing their health for the better but who doesn't know where to start, to start a food diary - then, you have the ability to look at what you are eating; calories, ratio of protein to carbohydrates and fats and so on. Once you have a baseline, you may also have already noticed an area that is in need of improvement. Start there, and go where your logic takes you, if you don't want to follow where my logic took me. I'm a lifelong learner, so I will often read multiple sources and come up with some version of my own recipe based on that research. That is exactly how I ended up on my path to regular fasting, probiotics, and a whole foods diet that leans toward the carnivore/keto side. It is also how I got interested in meditation, hydrogen water, grounding and any other health kick I might be interested in.

Experimenting with various diets and maintaining a diary of your results can be an enlightening journey toward better health and well-being. I can't encourage you enough to give it a try – you never know what you will learn!

The Quest for Optimal Nutrition:

- Our bodies are unique, and what works for one person may not work for another. Experimenting with different diets allows you to discover what truly nourishes you.
- Consider trying popular diets like keto, paleo, Mediterranean, vegan, or intermittent fasting. Each has its principles and potential benefits.

Keeping a Diet Diary:

- Start by creating a simple diary or digital log. Record what you eat, portion sizes, meal times, and any relevant observations (e.g., energy levels, mood, digestion).
- Be honest and detailed. Include snacks, beverages, and even emotional triggers for eating.

Tracking Results:

- After a week or two on a specific diet, assess how you feel. Are you more energetic? Less bloated? Sleeping better?
- Note any changes in weight, skin appearance, mental clarity, or digestive comfort.

Identifying Patterns:

- Over time, patterns emerge. Maybe you thrive on a plant-based diet, or perhaps you feel better with occasional meat.
- Pay attention to cravings, hunger cues, and emotional triggers. These insights guide your choices.

Adjustments and Adaptations:

- Diets aren't static. Adapt based on your body's signals. If something isn't working, tweak it.
- Gradually reintroduce foods you eliminated to see how your body responds.

Mindful Eating:

- Mindfulness matters. Savor each bite, listen to your body, and eat with intention.
- A diet diary helps you become more mindful of your food choices.

Long-Term Sustainability:

- Aim for a diet that aligns with your lifestyle and values. Sustainability matters more than short-term results.
- Remember, consistency over time yields the most significant impact.

In summary, your diet diary becomes a compass, guiding you toward optimal nutrition. It's not about perfection; it's about understanding what fuels your unique system.

12

Understanding Evolutionary Health

The sources I've relied on to shape my current program are deeply rooted in understanding how our bodies evolved and what our optimal diet and lifestyle might look like. Medical studies, evolutionary biology, and nutritional research all suggest that a diet low in processed foods, combined with practices like fasting and maintaining gut health, aligns well with our genetic makeup.

Our bodies carry an ancient blueprint—a genetic heritage shaped by millions of years of evolution. As we delve into the sources that inform our current health practices, we can see connections with our ancient ancestors, and the different struggles they faced. For example, starvation due to scarcity was much more likely to be a problem for our earliest ancestors than obesity due to excess. As a result, it makes sense that we should be efficient in storing any excess calories for those times of scarcity. The vast majority of us are unlikely to have to deal with a total lack of food. We struggle more with making healthy choices for the types and amount of food we consume.

Medical Studies: Bridging Science and Experience

- Modern medicine provides a lens through which we examine health. Rigorous studies dissect diseases, treatments, and preventive measures.
- Yet, medical science also acknowledges that our bodies evolved in vastly different environments. Our genes remember the savannas, forests, and riverbanks where our ancestors roamed.

Evolutionary Biology: Rewinding the Tape of Time

- Evolutionary biologists study fossils, DNA, and comparative anatomy. They piece together our evolutionary journey.
- Our distant forebears were hunter-gatherers—nimble, adaptable, and attuned to their surroundings. Their diets consisted of whole foods—wild plants, game, and seasonal fruits.

Nutritional Research: Decoding the Optimal Diet

- Nutritional science investigates macronutrients, micronutrients, and their impact on health.
- Researchers explore ancestral diets—the Paleolithic era, for instance. What did our predecessors eat? How did their bodies respond?
- The consensus emerges: Processed foods—laden with refined sugars, trans fats, and additives—deviate from our genetic expectations.

The Low-Processed Diet: A Return to Roots

- Our optimal diet mirrors the past. It's a symphony of fresh vegetables, fruits, lean proteins, and healthy fats.
- Processed foods—those alien to our ancestors—trigger inflammation, disrupt gut microbiota, and strain metabolic pathways.
- By minimizing processed foods, we honor our genetic legacy.

Fasting: Echoes of Scarcity and Resilience

- Fasting isn't new; it's ancient wisdom. Our ancestors faced feast and famine cycles.
- Intermittent fasting taps into our resilience. It resets metabolic processes, enhances autophagy (cellular cleanup), and promotes longevity.
- Fasting aligns with our evolutionary memory of scarcity and adaptation.

Gut Health: The Microbial Symphony Within

- Our gut microbiome—a bustling community of trillions of microbes—craves diversity.
- Fermented foods, fiber, and prebiotics nourish our gut. They echo the plant-based diets of our ancestors.
- A healthy gut supports digestion, immunity, and even mental well-being.

In conclusion, our bodies hum to an ancient melody. By embracing whole foods, fasting wisely, and nurturing our gut, we harmonize with our genetic makeup. As we tread this path, we honor the whispers of our ancestors—their resilience, wisdom, and survival instincts.

13

Psychological & Emotional Health

Weight loss is not just a physical journey but a psychological one too. The impact of self-perception, societal pressure, and emotional well-being cannot be understated. Throughout this journey, I have rediscovered the importance of a positive mindset and self-compassion. Understanding and addressing the emotional triggers that led to overeating or poor dietary choices was essential in maintaining my progress and fostering a healthier relationship with food.

Weight loss is a multifaceted expedition—one that transcends mere physical changes. As we embark on this path, we find ourselves navigating the intricate landscape of our minds and emotions. Let's delve into the psychological dimensions of this transformative journey:

The Inner Terrain: Navigating Self-Perception and Societal Pressures

Self-Perception: The Mirror Within

- Our perception of self profoundly influences our actions. When we view ourselves through a critical lens, it colors our choices.
- Weight loss often begins with a shift in self-perception. We learn to see beyond the numbers on a scale—to recognize our inherent worth and potential.

Societal Pressure: The Silent Chorus

- Society whispers expectations into our ears—the ideal body, the perfect shape. These whispers echo in dressing rooms, magazine covers, and social media feeds.
- The pressure to conform can be suffocating. Yet, we reclaim our power by questioning these norms and defining our own paths.

Emotional Well-Being: The Heart's Balance

- Our emotions intertwine with our eating habits. Stress, boredom, loneliness—they all find solace in food.
- Acknowledging our emotional triggers is liberating. We learn to nourish not just our bodies but also our hearts.

The Compass of Mindset and Self-Compassion

Positive Mindset: The North Star

- A positive mindset isn't blind optimism; it's resilience. It's the belief that setbacks are stepping stones, not roadblocks.
- When we face plateaus or slip-ups, a positive mindset whispers, "You're still moving forward."

Self-Compassion: The Gentle Guide

- We're often kinder to others than to ourselves. Self-compassion flips the script.
- It says, "You're human. You stumble, but you rise. You deserve love and understanding."

Emotional Triggers: Unmasking the Culprits

- Why did we reach for that extra cookie? What void were we trying to fill?
- By unraveling emotional triggers, we reclaim control. We find healthier ways to cope.

In this psychological odyssey, we learn that weight loss isn't just about shedding pounds; it's about shedding old beliefs, fears, and self-imposed limitations. So, as we step forward, let's carry self-compassion as our lantern and positive mindset as our compass.

14

Building a Support System

aving a supportive network has been invaluable. Sharing my experiences with friends, family, and online communities has provided encouragement and accountability. It's incredible how sharing stories and strategies can build camaraderie and motivation. For anyone embarking on a similar journey, I highly recommend finding a supportive group—whether local or online—that aligns with your goals.

Building Bridges: The Power of Supportive Networks

Embarking on a transformative journey—be it weight loss, personal growth, or creative pursuits—can feel like navigating uncharted waters. Yet, within this vast expanse, we discover the lighthouses that guide us—the supportive networks that illuminate our path. Let's explore how these connections shape our voyage:

Friends and Family: Anchors of Encouragement

- Our loved ones become our cheerleaders. They celebrate our victories, lend a listening ear during setbacks, and remind us of our resilience.
- Sharing our experiences with them creates a tapestry of understanding. Their empathy fuels our determination.

Online Communities: Virtual Campfires

- In the digital age, online communities serve as gathering places. Here, we find kindred spirits who've walked similar paths.
- These forums buzz with shared stories, vulnerability, and practical strategies. We learn from others' triumphs and pitfalls.

Encouragement and Accountability: Twin Sails

- Encouragement lifts our spirits. It whispers, "You're not alone." It nudges us forward when doubt creeps in.
- Accountability, like a compass, keeps us on course. When we commit to our goals publicly, we honor that commitment.

Camaraderie and Motivation: The Wind in Our Sails

- Camaraderie emerges from shared struggles. It's the nod of recognition—the "I've been there too."
- Motivation thrives in this ecosystem. We witness others' progress, and it fuels our own.

Finding Your Tribe: Local or Online

- Seek out your tribe—a group that resonates with your aspirations. It could be a local fitness class, a writing circle, or an online forum.
- Together, you'll weather storms, celebrate sunrises, and exchange maps to uncharted territories.

In the symphony of support, we find harmony. So, to fellow travelers, I echo the sentiment: Find your network, weave your stories, and let camaraderie be your compass.

15

Exercise and Movement

While diet and fasting have played a crucial role in my weight loss, incorporating regular physical activity has been equally important in supporting my overall health, if not my weight loss goals. I started with small, manageable goals, like walking and light stretching. Gradually, I've added more structured exercise routines, including strength training and yoga. These activities improve muscle tone, flexibility, and mental health.

Exercise After Menopause: Nurturing Well-Being

Cardiovascular Health: A Strong Heartbeat

Why It Matters: Declining estrogen during menopause affects metabolic function. Regular exercise supports cardiovascular health.
Benefits:

- **Heart Protection:** Exercise reduces the risk of heart disease, high blood pressure, and stroke.
- **Weight Management:** Physical activity helps maintain a healthy

weight, which is vital for heart health.

Bone Strength: Building Resilience

Why It Matters: Menopause leads to bone loss, increasing the risk of fractures and osteoporosis.
Benefits:

- **Weight-Bearing Activities:** Walking, running, and strength training preserve bone mass.
- **Fracture Prevention:** Exercise reduces the likelihood of fractures by maintaining bone density.

Mood and Mental Clarity: The Endorphin Boost

Why It Matters: Hormonal changes can impact mood and cognitive function.
Benefits:

- **Endorphins:** Exercise releases endorphins—natural mood enhancers.
- **Stress Reduction:** Physical activity combats stress, anxiety, and depression.

Balance and Flexibility: Preventing Falls

Why It Matters: Falls become riskier with age due to bone fragility.
Benefits:

- **Balance Training:** Yoga, tai chi, and balance exercises improve stability.

- **Fall Prevention:** Enhanced balance reduces the risk of falls and related injuries.

Weight Management: Avoiding Unwanted Pounds

Why It Matters: Many women experience weight gain during menopause.
  Benefits:

- **Caloric Burn:** Exercise helps maintain a healthy weight.
- **Metabolism Boost:** Regular physical activity supports efficient metabolism.

Overall Well-Being: The Holistic Approach

Why It Matters: Menopause isn't just physical—it's emotional and mental too.
  Benefits:

- **Quality of Life:** Exercise improves sleep, energy levels, and overall well-being.
- **Community and Connection:** Group activities foster camaraderie and motivation.

Remember, exercise isn't a chore—it's an investment in your health. Whether it's a brisk walk, a dance class, or weight training, find what brings you joy. Consult your healthcare provider to tailor an exercise plan that suits your needs.

16

Overcoming Plateaus

Like any weight loss journey, I encountered plateaus that tested my patience and resolve. These stagnant periods were challenging, but by focusing on the broader picture and experimenting with slight adjustments—whether in my fasting schedule, exercise routine, or dietary intake—I was able to navigate through them. Understanding that plateaus are part of the process helped keep discouragement at bay and motivated me to persist.

Navigating Plateaus: The Steady Climb

Weight loss, like any journey, isn't a straight path—it's a winding trail with unexpected plateaus. These moments test our mettle, but they also reveal our resilience. Let's explore how to conquer these weight loss plateaus:

The Plateau Paradox: When Progress Pauses

- **What It Feels Like:** Imagine climbing a mountain. Suddenly, the slope levels off. You're still moving, but the peak seems elusive.
- **Why Plateaus Occur:**
- Our bodies adapt. What worked initially becomes less effective.
- Water retention, hormonal shifts, and muscle gain can mask fat loss.
- **The Mental Game:** Plateaus mess with our minds. Doubt creeps in. We wonder if we've hit a dead end.

Zoom Out: The Broader Picture

- **Shift Perspective:** Instead of fixating on the plateau, zoom out. Look at the entire landscape—the progress you've made.
- **Non-Scale Victories:** Celebrate non-scale victories—more energy, better sleep, improved mood. These matter too.

Experimentation: Tinkering with the Formula

- **Fasting Schedule:** Adjust your fasting window. Maybe extend it or change the timing.
- **Exercise Routine:** Surprise your muscles. Vary workouts—try HIIT, dance, or outdoor activities.
- **Dietary Intake:** Tweak macros. Add more protein, reduce carbs, or explore new foods.

Mind the Mindset: Keep Discouragement at Bay

- **Normalize Plateaus:** They're part of the process. Every successful journey encounters them.
- **Patience and Persistence:** Remind yourself that persistence pays off. You're not stuck; you're recalibrating.

Motivation Rekindled: The Fire Within

- **Visualize Success:** Imagine reaching your goal. Feel it—the energy, confidence, and vitality.
- **Remember Why:** Why did you start this journey? Reconnect with that initial spark.

Community and Accountability: Share the Climb

- **Supportive Network:** Lean on friends, family, or online communities. Share your plateau woes.
- **Accountability Partner:** Find someone who cheers you on and gently nudges you forward.

Remember, plateaus aren't roadblocks; they're pit stops. Adjust your gear, catch your breath, and keep climbing. The peak awaits.

17

Sharing Knowledge and Giving Back

One of the most rewarding aspects of my journey has been the opportunity to share what I've learned with others. Whether through social media, local support groups, or casual conversations, I've been able to provide guidance and encouragement to those facing similar struggles. Giving back and helping others find their own paths to health has enriched my experience and reinforced my commitment to this lifestyle.

Passing the Torch: Sharing Wisdom on the Journey

In the tapestry of our personal transformations, there lies a thread of generosity—a desire to illuminate the path for others. As I reflect on my weight loss journey, I find solace in the moments when I extended my hand to fellow travelers. Here's why sharing our insights matters:

Social Media: A Digital Campfire

- **Why It Works:** Social media platforms connect us across distances. We share snippets of our lives, victories, and struggles.
- **My Role:** I've become a torchbearer—posting about breakthroughs, recipes, and setbacks. Others find solace in these virtual campfires.

Local Support Groups: The Circle of Empathy

- **Why It Matters:** Face-to-face interactions create bonds. Local groups—whether fitness classes or wellness circles—become our sanctuaries.
- **My Contribution:** I've sat in those circles, listened, and shared. We swap tips, recipes, and stories. We nod, knowing we're not alone.

Casual Conversations: Seeds of Change

- **Why They Count:** Casual chats ripple outward. A coffee chat with a friend, a chat at the grocery store—it all matters.
- **My Words:** I've whispered encouragement, debunked myths, and sparked curiosity. Sometimes, a single sentence alters someone's course.

The Ripple Effect: Enriching Our Own Journey

- **Why It's Rewarding:** When we give, we receive. Sharing wisdom isn't a one-way street.
- **My Heart's Echo:** Helping others find their paths reinforces my commitment. It's a reminder that our journeys intersect, intertwine, and amplify.

Legacy of Light: Passing the Torch

- **Why It's Timeless:** Our ancestors shared stories around fires. We continue that tradition—digitally, in person, through whispers.
- **My Hope:** Those I've guided will, in turn, guide others. The torch passes—a legacy of resilience, compassion, and health.

So, fellow traveler, let's keep sharing. Whether it's a tweet, a hug, or a handwritten note, our words ripple through time

18

Reflecting On Long-Term Sustainability

Sustainability is at the core of my approach. The changes I've implemented are ones I can envision maintaining for the rest of my life. Unlike past attempts focused on short-term gains, this journey is about creating a lasting, healthy lifestyle. The balance I've struck allows me to enjoy occasional indulgences without guilt, knowing that my foundational habits will support continued health and weight maintenance.

In the tapestry of transformation, sustainability weaves the strongest threads. Unlike fleeting fads, my journey is anchored in enduring choices—ones that harmonize with life's rhythm. Here's why sustainability is my compass:

Vision Beyond the Horizon: A Lifetime Commitment

- **Why It Matters:** Short-term gains fade like shooting stars. I seek constellations—the enduring glow.
- **My Approach:** Every change I make is a pledge—a lifelong

commitment. I envision myself thriving in my 80s, still savoring vibrant health.

The Art of Balance: Nourishing Body and Soul

- **Why Balance Is Key:** Extremes burn out. Sustainability lies in moderation.
- **My Equation:** I indulge occasionally—desserts, celebrations—but my daily canvas is painted with whole foods, movement, and mindfulness.

Guilt-Free Pleasures: Savoring the Present

- **Why Guilt Has No Place:** Guilt corrodes joy. Instead, I savor indulgences mindfully.
- **My Mantra:** A slice of cake isn't a sin; it's a celebration. Guilt-free, I move forward.

Foundational Habits: The Bedrock of Health

- **Why They Matter:** Foundations withstand storms. My habits—daily walks, nourishing meals, restful sleep—are bedrock.
- **My Assurance:** Even during plateaus or setbacks, these habits cradle me.

Legacy of Wellness: Passing It On

- **Why I Share:** Like a seasoned gardener, I plant seeds. I share recipes, tips, and encouragement.
- **My Joy:** When someone says, "Your journey inspired me," I know I've sown well.

So, fellow traveler, let's walk this sustainable path. May our choices echo through generations—a legacy of health, joy, and balance.

53

19

Embracing Change

Change can be daunting, but embracing it has been essential in achieving my health goals. I've learned to be flexible and adaptive, welcoming new practices and discarding those that no longer serve me. This dynamic approach has kept the process interesting and manageable, allowing me to stay motivated and engaged.

The Dance of Transformation

Change—the chameleon of life—slips into our routines, uninvited yet inevitable. It wears many masks: fear, uncertainty, and possibility. As I tread the path toward health, I've learned to waltz with change—to let it lead, even when my feet stumble. Here's why embracing change has been my compass:

The Daunting Threshold: Fear and Invitation

- **Why It Matters:** Change knocks on our doors, disguised as a challenge. It whispers, "Are you ready?"
- **My Response:** I've flung open the door. Fear and curiosity coexist.

Change isn't an intruder; it's an invitation.

Flexibility and Adaptability: The Dance Steps

- **Why They Matter:** Rigid routines crumble. Adaptability is my partner.
- **My Moves:**
- **Welcoming New Practices:** Intermittent fasting, mindful eating, yoga—I've invited them in.
- **Discarding Old Habits:** Farewell, mindless snacking and sedentary hours. You no longer serve me.

Dynamic Approach: The Ever-Adjusting Sails

- **Why It Keeps Me Afloat:** Life isn't static; neither is health. I adjust my sails.
- **My Toolbox:**
- **Tweaking Fasting Schedules:** Sometimes 16:8, sometimes 14:10. Adaptation is my secret sauce.
- **Exploring Workouts:** From brisk walks to HIIT, I keep my muscles guessing.
- **Culinary Adventures:** New recipes, seasonal produce—I savor the variety.

Intriguing Process: The Novelty Factor

- **Why It Engages Me:** Monotony breeds apathy. Novelty sparks curiosity.
- **My Playground:** Change keeps the journey interesting. I'm not on a treadmill; I'm exploring uncharted trails.

Motivation and Engagement: The Fire Within

- **Why I Stay Aflame:** Change fuels motivation. It's the wind beneath my wings.
- **My Mantra:** "What's next?" I ask, eyes alight. The answer propels me forward.

So, fellow dancer, let's sway with change. It's not a foe; it's our partner—a rhythm we learn, unlearn, and relearn.

20

The Emotional Rewards

The emotional rewards of this journey are immense. Beyond the physical transformations, the sense of accomplishment, increased self-esteem, and better emotional health have been profound. I feel more confident, comfortable in my own skin, and empowered to face life's challenges. The improvements in my mood and overall outlook on life have been as significant as the physical benefits.

Brushstrokes of Transformation

In the quiet chambers of change, emotions whisper. They're the hues that color our journey—a canvas where victories and setbacks blend. As I navigate this labyrinth, I find that the emotional palette is as vivid as the physical shifts:

Sense of Accomplishment: A Symphony of Small Wins

- **Why It Resonates:** Each choice—each step—is a note. The symphony isn't just the grand finale; it's the crescendo of daily efforts.
- **My Melody:** I hum it softly—the tune of progress, resilience, and quiet triumphs.

Increased Self-Esteem: A Portrait of Strength

- **Why It Captures:** Weight loss isn't vanity; it's self-love. As the mirror reflects change, so does my perception.
- **My Reflection:** I see courage in my eyes. My esteem blooms, petal by petal.

Better Emotional Health: The Healing Balm

- **Why It Soothes:** Emotional weight—like rain-soaked soil—can drown or nourish.
- **My Rituals:**
- **Mindfulness:** I sip tea mindfully, savoring warmth.
- **Gratitude:** I collect moments—the sun's kiss, a friend's laughter.
- **Self-Compassion:** I cradle my heart, whispering, "You're enough."

Confidence and Comfort: Tailored Garments

- **Why They Fit:** I wear confidence like a bespoke suit. It's tailored to my journey.
- **My Stride:** I walk unafraid, comfortable in my skin. Confidence is my second heartbeat.

Empowerment: The Sword of Resolve

- **Why It's Forged:** Life's dragons—challenges—require armor. Empowerment is my sword.
- **My Battle Cry:** "I can face this." And I do, with grace and fire.

Mood and Outlook: Sunrises Within

- **Why They Illuminate:** The sun rises not only in the sky but also in our hearts.
- **My Forecast:** Brighter days ahead. Optimism is my compass.

So, fellow artist, let's paint with emotion. Our strokes—bold, delicate, imperfect—compose the masterpiece of transformation.

21

Empowerment Through Knowledge

Knowledge is power. The more I learned about health, nutrition, and the human body, the more empowered I felt to make informed decisions that align with my goals. Continuous learning and staying updated with the latest research have been crucial elements of my success.

In the labyrinth of health, knowledge isn't just a lantern—it's a compass, a map, and a guiding star. As I tread this path, I've discovered that the pursuit of understanding is as vital as the steps I take. Here's why knowledge has become my most potent ally:

The Alchemical Transformation: From Ignorance to Empowerment

- **Why It Matters:** Ignorance breeds vulnerability. Knowledge, on the other hand, is the elixir that transforms uncertainty into resolve.
- **My Journey:** I've delved into textbooks, research papers, and podcasts. Each discovery—whether about macronutrients, gut microbiota, or circadian rhythms—has fortified my resolve.

Nutrition: Decoding the Culinary Glyphs

- **Why It Nourishes:** Food isn't just sustenance; it's a language. Nutrients speak to our cells, orchestrating vitality or dissonance.
- **My Lexicon:** I've studied labels, dissected ingredients, and deciphered the hieroglyphs of vitamins and minerals. Each choice at the grocery store is a sentence in my health narrative.

Human Body: The Living Canvas

- **Why It Inspires:** Our bodies are masterpieces—biological canvases painted with intricate strokes. Muscles ripple, bones scaffold, and neurons fire.
- **My Palette:** I mix colors—endocrine pathways, immune responses, and neural networks. The canvas breathes.

Latest Research: The Quill of Progress

- **Why It's My Quiver:** Science evolves. Research is our time-traveler—unearthing ancient wisdom, debunking myths.
- **My Rituals:**
- **PubMed Quests:** I explore studies—intermittent fasting, sleep

hygiene, epigenetics.

- **Health Podcasts:** Voices of experts—like whispers in the wind.

Empowerment: The Sword of Choice

- **Why It's Forged:** Knowledge isn't passive; it's a sword. I wield it—against misinformation, against complacency.
- **My Battle Cry:** "I choose health." And I do, with conviction.

Legacy of Learning: Passing the Torch

- **Why It's Timeless:** Our ancestors shared stories around fires. We continue that tradition—digitally, in person, through whispers.
- **My Hope:** Those I've guided will, in turn, guide others. The torch passes—a legacy of curiosity, resilience, and health.

So, fellow seeker, let's unravel this scroll. Knowledge isn't power; it's empowerment—the spark that ignites our journey.

22

Building New Habits

uilding new habits requires time and patience. Initially, some of the changes felt daunting and unnatural, but with persistence, they have become second nature. Establishing a routine that includes regular exercise, mindful eating, adequate sleep, and stress management has created a solid foundation for lifelong health.

In the quiet atelier of transformation, I wield my brushes—time and patience—as I sculpt new habits. The canvas is blank, and the strokes feel tentative, like whispers against the wind. But with each deliberate mark, the daunting becomes familiar, the unnatural—organic.

The Clay of Persistence: Patience as My Chisel

- **Why It Matters:** Habits aren't carved in a day. They're chiseled—slowly, deliberately.
- **My Studio:** I sit—brush in hand—shaping routines. The clay yields, then resists. I persist.

The Palette of Adaptation: From Daunting to Second Nature

- **Why It Transforms:** Change is a palette—colors blending, shifting. At first, the hues clash.
- **My Mixes:**
- **Morning Runs:** Daunting at dawn, now a sunrise ritual.
- **Mindful Meals:** Unnatural forks become mindful bites.
- **Sleep Rituals:** Unfamiliar bedtime routines now cradle dreams.

The Blueprint of Balance: A Routine's Architecture

- **Why It Holds:** Habits need scaffolding—exercise, nourishment, rest, and serenity.
- **My Blueprint:**
- **Exercise:** Brushstrokes of movement—yoga, walks, dance.
- **Mindful Eating:** Each bite—a stroke of intention.
- **Sleep Sanctuary:** Pillows cradle dreams; rituals dim the lights.
- **Stress Management:** Breaths—like gentle strokes—calm the canvas.

The Masterpiece of Health: A Lifelong Legacy

- **Why It's My Magnum Opus:** Habits aren't just strokes; they're the entire canvas.
- **My Signature:** I sign—commitment, resilience, and whispers of well-being.

The Gallery of Tomorrow: A Solid Foundation

- **Why It Endures:** Habits echo through time. They're the gallery—where health hangs.
- **My Invitation:** Visitors—future selves—will admire this foundation. It's their legacy too.

So, fellow artist, let's sculpt. Our habits—bold, delicate, imperfect—compose the masterpiece of lifelong health.

23

Finding Joy in the Journey

Finding joy in the journey rather than focusing solely on the end goal has made the process fulfilling. Celebrating small victories, enjoying healthier foods, and finding pleasure in new forms of exercise have all contributed to a positive and enriching experience.

As an artist of well-being, I've learned that the journey isn't just a means to an end—it's a masterpiece in progress. The brushstrokes matter—the small victories, the mindful bites, the rhythmic steps. Here's why finding joy in the journey has transformed my canvas:

The Palette of Small Victories: Celebrating Each Hue

- **Why It Illuminates:** Life isn't a single grand finale; it's a series of vignettes. Each victory—a brushstroke—adds depth.
- **My Gallery:** I hang these moments—finishing a morning run, resisting that sugary temptation, hitting a personal best. Each frame whispers, "You're on the right path."

Healthier Foods: A Flavorful Palette

- **Why It Nourishes:** Food isn't just sustenance; it's a symphony. Kale crunches, berries burst, and quinoa dances.
- **My Tastings:** I explore—farmers' markets, spice aisles, recipe books. Each bite is a note—a harmony of nutrients and pleasure.

New Forms of Exercise: The Choreography of Joy

- **Why It Moves Me:** Exercise isn't punishment; it's choreography. Yoga flows, dance steps, trail runs—they're my dances with gravity.
- **My Playlist:** I sync—heartbeats, playlists, and the rhythm of my breath. Each move is a brushstroke on my canvas of vitality.

The End Goal: A Hidden Horizon

- **Why It Shifts:** The summit isn't the sole vista; it's the entire ascent. The end goal—like a distant mountain peak—guides me, but the valleys, the wildflowers, and the sunsets—they're my treasures.

Enriching Experience: The Artist's Signature

- **Why It Matters:** The journey isn't a draft; it's the final piece. I sign it—gratitude, resilience, and the joy of becoming.
- **My Brush:** It glides—over setbacks, over breakthroughs. Each stroke is a whisper: "This is life."

So, fellow artist, let's paint joy. Our canvas—bold, delicate, imperfect—holds the hues of fulfillment.

$$24$$

Real Life Application

The principles and practices I've adopted are integrated into my daily life seamlessly. They are not rigid rules but guidelines that allow for flexibility and adaptation. Whether traveling, socializing, or dealing with unexpected events, I can apply these principles in a way that supports my health without feeling restricted or stressed.

Principles, Not Shackles

In the symphony of well-being, rigidity is a discordant note. As I compose my daily life, I've chosen principles over rules—guidelines that sway with the rhythm of existence. Here's why this fluidity has become my anthem:

The Dance of Integration: Principles as Choreography

- **Why It Resonates:** Life isn't a solo; it's a pas de deux. Principles—like graceful steps—integrate seamlessly.
- **My Choreography:**

- **Morning Rituals:** A pirouette of hydration, a plié of gratitude.
- **Nutrition:** A waltz of colors—leafy greens, vibrant fruits.
- **Movement:** A tango of walks, yoga, and spontaneous dances.

Flexibility: The Melody of Adaptation

- **Why It Harmonizes:** Rigid rules snap; principles sway. They're the jazz improvisations—the syncopated rhythms.
- **My Score:** I play—traveling, socializing, navigating life's crescendos. Principles adjust—the tempo quickens, then slows.

Traveling Light: Principles in My Suitcase

- **Why They Fit:** Suitcases bulge with rules; backpacks carry principles. They're lightweight, adaptable.
- **My Packing List:**
- **Mindful Eating:** Local flavors, portion awareness.
- **Movement:** Urban hikes, impromptu stretches.
- **Rest:** Jet-lagged naps, starlit slumbers.

Unexpected Events: The Improvised Symphony

- **Why It Resonates:** Life throws cymbals—unexpected events. Principles—like jazz solos—improvise.
- **My Solo:** I riff—deep breaths during traffic jams, gratitude when plans unravel.

Stress-Free Notes: Principles, Not Shackles

- **Why They Soothe:** Principles don't strangle; they cradle. Stress dissipates; joy crescendos.
- **My Anthem:** "I choose health." And I do, with ease.

So, fellow composer, let's harmonize. Our principles—fluid, adaptable, alive—compose the symphony of well-being.

25

Addressing Skepticism and Misinformation

One of the challenges I've faced is dealing with skepticism and misinformation about the methods I'm using. In a world filled with diet fads and conflicting advice, it's crucial to discern credible sources and make informed decisions. Addressing these misconceptions head-on and sharing evidence-based insights have been integral in fostering a supportive and informed community around me.

In the labyrinth of wellness, I've encountered skeptics who raise their eyebrows at my unconventional methods. They tilt their heads, questioning my choices—fasting, meditation, and the mystical hydrogen water. In a cacophony of diet fads and contradictory counsel, I've learned that discernment is my compass.

"But isn't fasting dangerous?" they ask, their eyes wide with concern. I smile, unruffled. I've delved into research, separating wheat from chaff. Fasting, when done mindfully, can rejuvenate cells, boost autophagy, and re-calibrate metabolic rhythms. It's not deprivation; it's liberation.

"Hydrogen water? Sounds like snake oil!" they scoff. I nod, understanding their skepticism. Yet, studies whisper secrets: molecular hydrogen as an antioxidant, scavenging free radicals, dancing with inflammation.

I sip my effervescent elixir, knowing its silent magic.

And misinformation? Ah, the hydra-headed beast! I wield my sword—anecdotes, peer-reviewed papers, and expert interviews. I share, not preach. I've seen eyes widen, minds shift. The community around me blossoms—a garden of seekers, each tending to their own well-being.

In this world of noise, I've become a curator. I sift through the sands of advice, seeking pearls of wisdom. I embrace consistency, sustainability, and a positive mindset. My journey isn't dogma; it's fluid—a river carving its course.

So, let's navigate these waters together. Let's sip hydrogen-infused, sugar-free truth, fast from misinformation, and meditate on resilience and sustainability. And when skeptics raise their brows, we'll smile—a ripple of knowing. For we're not just seekers; we're torchbearers, illuminating the path toward vibrant living.

26

The Role of Healthcare Providers

Collaboration with healthcare providers has been an important aspect of my journey. Regular check-ups, consultations, and discussions about my progress and strategies have provided additional support and validation. Healthcare professionals can offer personalized advice and ensure that the chosen methods are safe and effective.

Consulting a healthcare professional before making any diet or lifestyle changes is crucial for several reasons:

Personalization and Safety:

- Healthcare providers consider your unique health history, existing conditions, and medications. They tailor recommendations to your specific needs.
- Some diets or lifestyle changes may interact with medications or exacerbate underlying health issues. A professional can guide you safely.

Evidence-Based Guidance:

- Healthcare professionals stay updated on the latest research and evidence. They can separate fads from proven strategies.
- Their advice is grounded in science, ensuring you make informed choices.

Avoiding Harmful Practices:

- Drastic diets or extreme fasting can harm your body. A professional helps you avoid dangerous practices.
- They guide gradual, sustainable changes that promote long-term health.

Monitoring Progress:

- Regular check-ins allow professionals to track your progress. They adjust recommendations as needed.
- Monitoring ensures you stay on track and address any setbacks promptly.

Emotional Support:

- Lifestyle changes can be challenging. Professionals provide emotional support and encouragement.
- They celebrate your victories and help you navigate obstacles.

Remember, your well-being is a collaborative effort. Consult a healthcare provider—it's an investment in your health journey!

Resources

A PA PsycNet. (n.d.). https://psycnet.apa.org/record/2003-03727-001

Book summary: The Compound Effect by Darren Hardy. (2020, November 12). James Clear. https://jamesclear.com/book-summaries/the-compound-effect

Boyers, L., & TanyaJoy/iStock/GettyImages. (2019, May 8). *The benefits of ketosis.* Livestrong.com. https://www.livestrong.com/article/503671-the-benefits-of-ketosis/

Brooks, S. (2020, November 10). *The 5 stages of fasting (And the benefits of each one).* Perfect Keto. https://perfectketo.com/the-5-stages-of-fasting/

Brown, B. (2022). *The gifts of imperfection: Let Go of Who You Think You're Supposed to Be and Embrace Who You Are.* Simon and Schuster.

Choosing Whole Foods for a Healthier You» Mayo Clinic Connect. (n.d.).

Mayo Clinic Connect. https://connect.mayoclinic.org/blog/weight-management-1/newsfeed-post/choosing-whole-foods-for-a-healthier-you/

Clear, J. (2020, February 4). *How to stop Procrastinating by using the "2-Minute Rule."* James Clear. https://jamesclear.com/how-to-stop-procrastinating

Clinic, C. (2024a, May 3). *6 tips for fasting safely.* Cleveland Clinic. https://health.clevelandclinic.org/tips-for-fasting-the-healthy-way

Clinic, C. (2024b, May 10). *How to break that frustrating Weight-Loss plateau.* Cleveland Clinic. https://health.clevelandclinic.org/weight-loss-plateau

Cordain, L., Eaton, S. B., Sebastian, A., Mann, N., Lindeberg, S., Watkins, B. A., O'Keefe, J. H., & Brand-Miller, J. (2005). Origins and evolution of the Western diet: health implications for the 21st century1,2. *the American Journal of Clinical Nutrition, 81*(2), 341–354. https://doi.org/10.1093/ajcn.81.2.341

Cpt, K. D. M. R. (2023, April 19). *What is ketosis, and is it healthy?* Healthline. https://www.healthline.com/nutrition/what-is-ketosis

Eaton, S. B., & Konner, M. (1985). Paleolithic nutrition: A consideration of its nature and current implications. *New England Journal of Medicine, 312*(5), 283–289.

Garone, S. (2024, May 28). *The impact of food additives on health: What you need to know.* EverydayHealth.com. https://www.everydayhealth.com/diet-nutrition/how-safe-are-food-preservatives/

Gladwell, M. (2008). *Outliers: The Story of Success*. Penguin UK.

Hardy, D. (2011). *The compound effect*. Vanguard Press.

Harvard Health. (2021, November 1). *Meditation for your health*. https://www.health.harvard.edu/mind-and-mood/meditation-for-your-health

Harvard Health. (2023, July 18). *The gut-brain connection*. https://www.health.harvard.edu/diseases-and-conditions/the-gut-brain-connection

Howland, J. (2018, January 3). *Mayo Clinic Minute: Lose weight with a food diary*. Mayo Clinic News Network. https://newsnetwork.mayoclinic.org/discussion/mayo-clinic-minute-lose-weight-with-a-food-diary/

Kotifani, A. (2020, June 2). Fasting for health and longevity: Nobel Prize winning research on cell aging. *Blue Zones*. https://www.bluezones.com/2018/10/fasting-for-health-and-longevity-nobel-prize-winning-research-on-cell-aging/

Ldn, K. D. M. M. R. (2019, January 31). *Why keep a food diary?* Harvard Health. https://www.health.harvard.edu/blog/why-keep-a-food-diary-2019013115855

Levine, B., & Klionsky, D. J. (2016). Autophagy wins the 2016 Nobel Prize in Physiology or Medicine: Breakthroughs in baker's yeast fuel advances in biomedical research. *Proceedings of the National Academy of Sciences of the United States of America, 114*(2), 201–205. https://doi.org/10.1073/pnas.1619876114

Neff, K. (2003). Self-Compassion: an alternative conceptualization of a healthy attitude toward oneself. *Self and Identity*, *2*(2), 85–101. https://doi.org/10.1080/15298860309032

O'Keefe, J. H., & Cordain, L. (2003). Cardiovascular disease resulting from a diet and lifestyle at odds with our paleolithic genome: How to become a 21st-century hunter-gatherer. *Mayo Clinic Proceedings*, *79*(1), 101–108.

Patterson, R. (2022, November 9). The power of consistency. *Forbes*. https://www.forbes.com/sites/forbescoachescouncil/2020/11/02/the-power-of-consistency/?sh=269f18a228c7

Proctor, L. M. (2016a). The National Institutes of Health Human Microbiome Project. *Seminars in Fetal & Neonatal Medicine*, *21*(6), 368–372. https://doi.org/10.1016/j.siny.2016.05.002

Professional, C. C. M. (n.d.). *Ketosis*. Cleveland Clinic. https://my.cleve landclinic.org/health/articles/24003-ketosis

Rd, R. a. M. (2023, September 22). *8 Health benefits of fasting, backed by science*. Healthline. https://www.healthline.com/nutrition/fasting-ben efits

Specialized Women's Health & Menopause | Cleveland Clinic. (n.d.). Cleveland Clinic. https://my.clevelandclinic.org/departments/obg yn-womens-health/depts/specialized-womens-health

Team, W. (2024, February 5). *Clean eating: How to begin a whole foods diet.* Shine365. https://shine365.marshfieldclinic.org/wellness/whole-foods-diet-tips/

The Nobel Prize in Physiology or Medicine 2016. (n.d.). NobelPrize.org. https://www.nobelprize.org/prizes/medicine/2016/press-release/

Why this Japanese scientist won a 2016 Nobel Prize in medicine for cell 'self-eating.' (2016, October 3). PBS NewsHour. https://www.pbs.org/news hour/science/japanese-scientist-won-nobel-prize-cell-sclf-eating

Yamut, T. J., RN. (2023, June 13). *Ketosis: symptoms, benefits, risks, and more.* Perfect Keto. https://perfectketo.com/what-is-ketosis/

www.ingramcontent.com/pod-product-compliance
Lightning Source LLC
Chambersburg PA
CBHW051832250726
48659CB00005B/1797